I AM A
V.I.P.
(VERY IMPORTANT PATIENT)

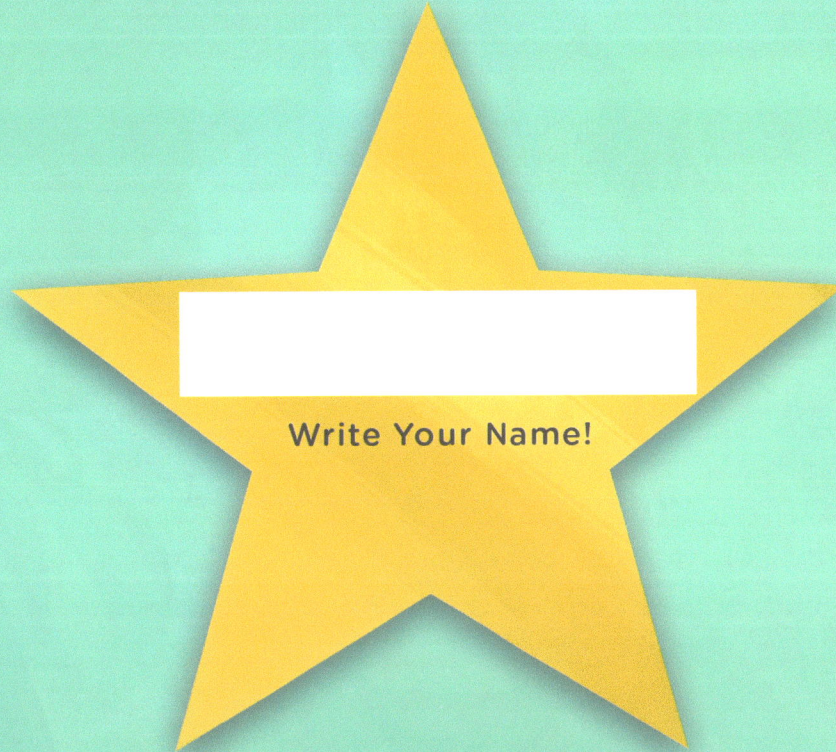

Write Your Name!

ISBN: 978-1-63110-374-2

A Product of V.I.P. Hospital Productions
www.viphospitalproductions.org
Design and Artwork by: Jillian Stiles

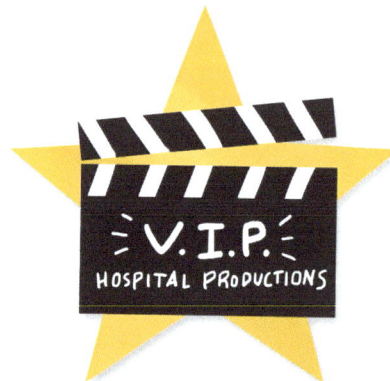

V.I.P. PASS

NAME

AGE

HAIR COLOR

EYE COLOR

Draw yourself!

Have an adult help you cut this out! ✂

Practice Your *Autograph*

Write your name **BIG + BOLD**

Write your name really small

Write your name with *Fancy Letters*

Write you name in your favorite **Color**

Write your name **backwards**

Create your own unique way!

Welcome to the Chinese Theater

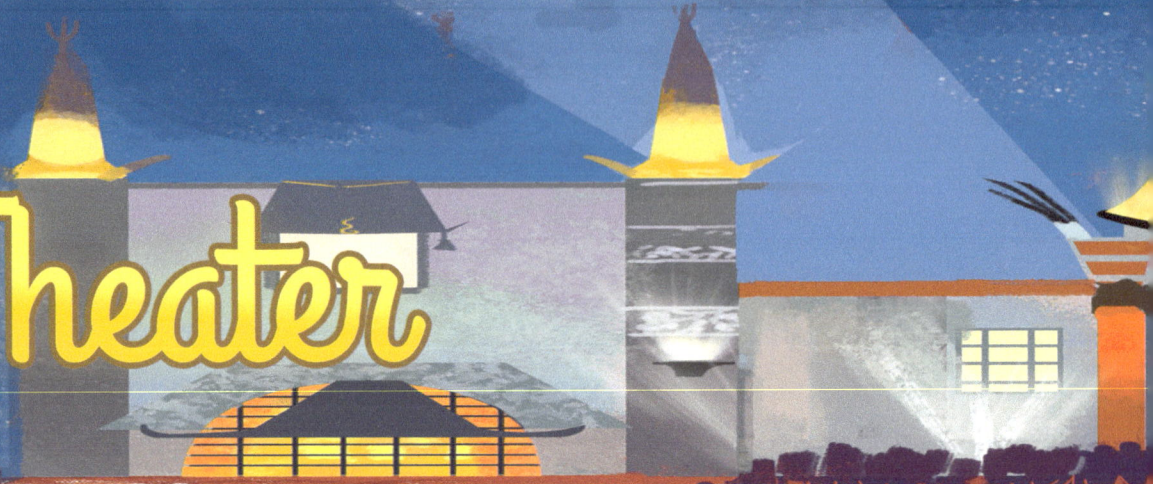

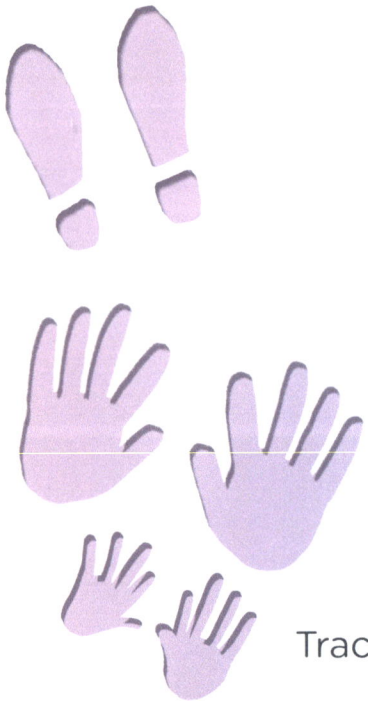

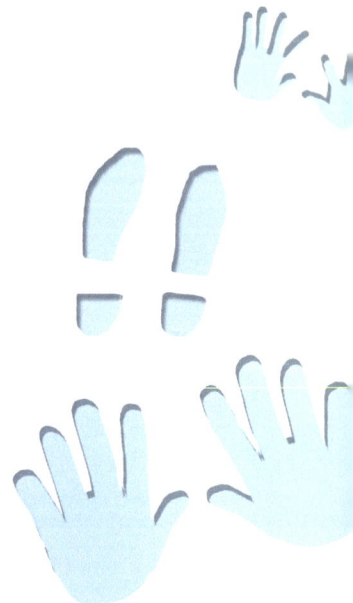

Trace your left hand and on each finger write one great thing about you!

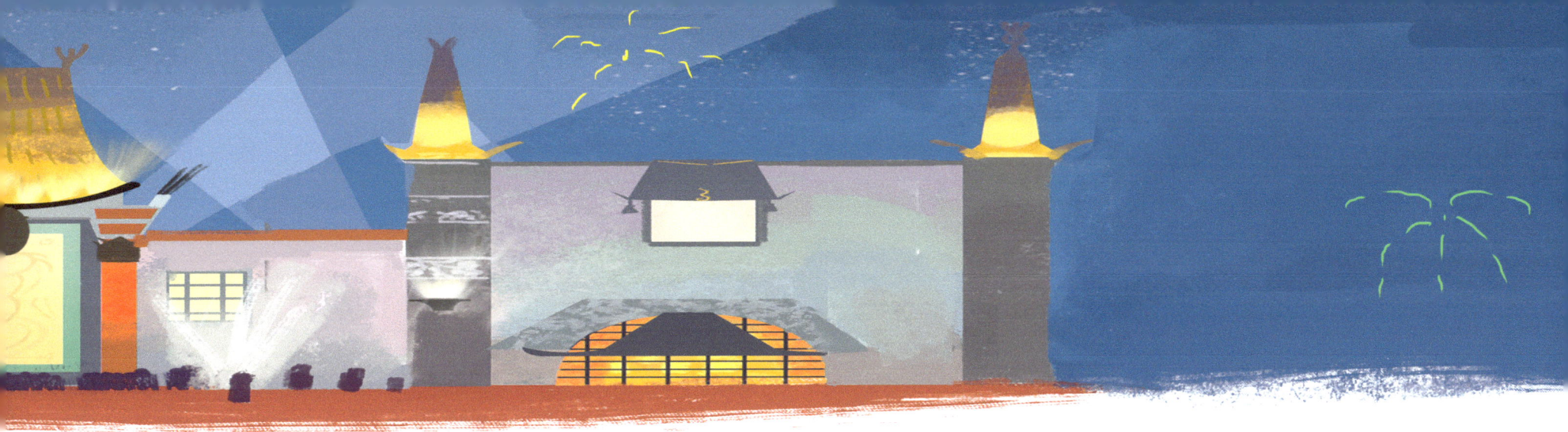

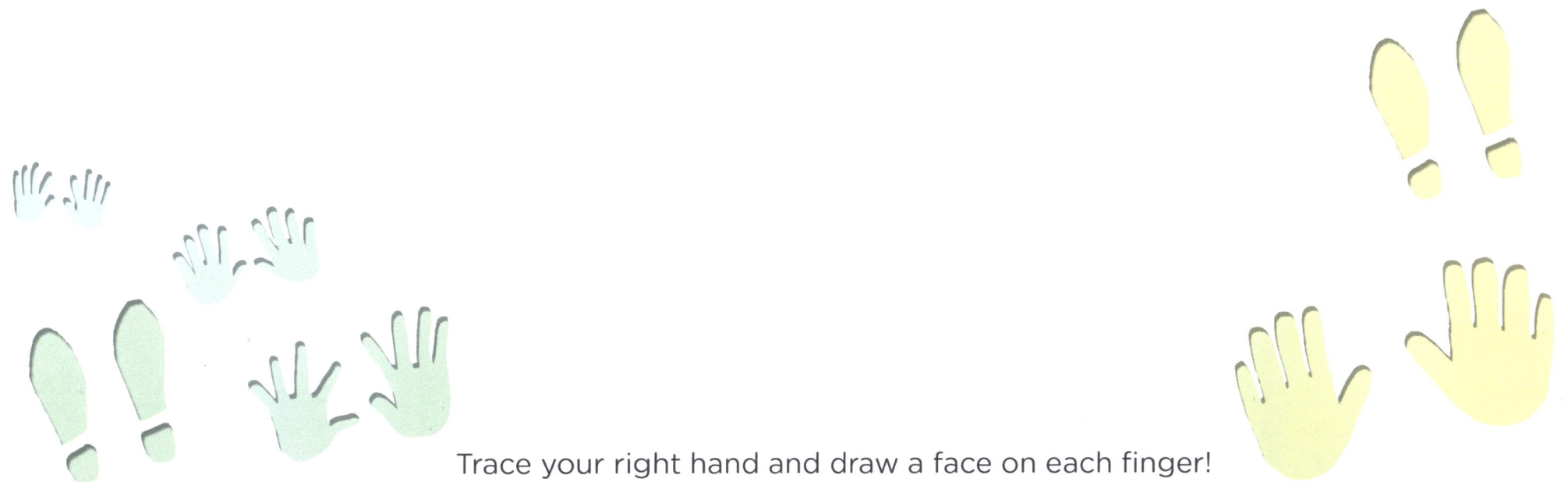

Trace your right hand and draw a face on each finger!

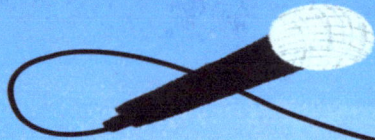

V.I.P. BIOGRAPHY

My full name:

Nickname:

My age:

The city and state I live in:

I one day hope to visit:

My special talents:

My favorite movie/T.V. Show:

My favorite book:

My favorite music or band:

My favorite animal:

My favorite subject in school:

My favorite color:

My favorite food:

Things I love:

Things I hate:

When I'm with my friends I like to:

DRAW A PICTURE OF YOU ON THE RED CARPET

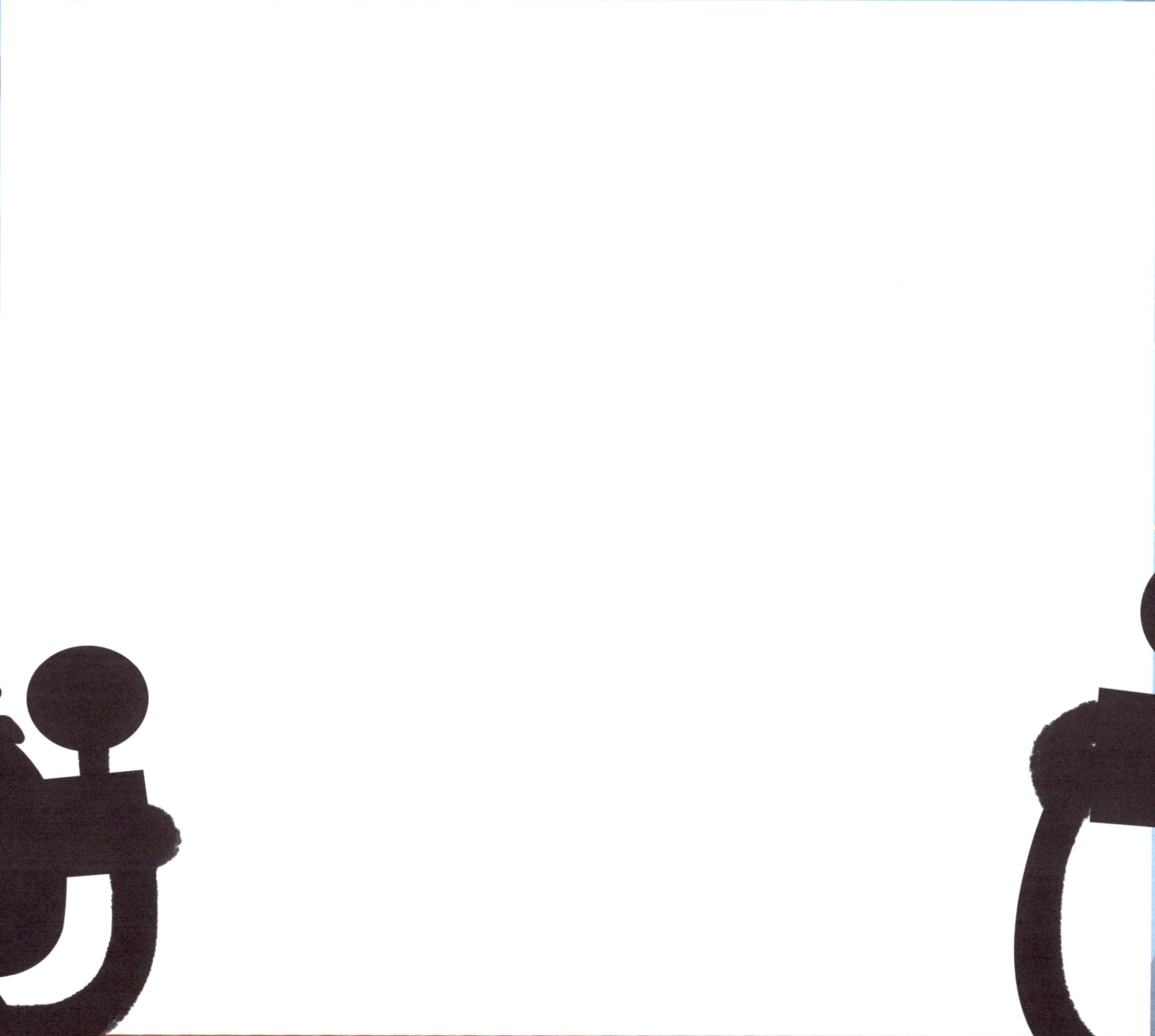

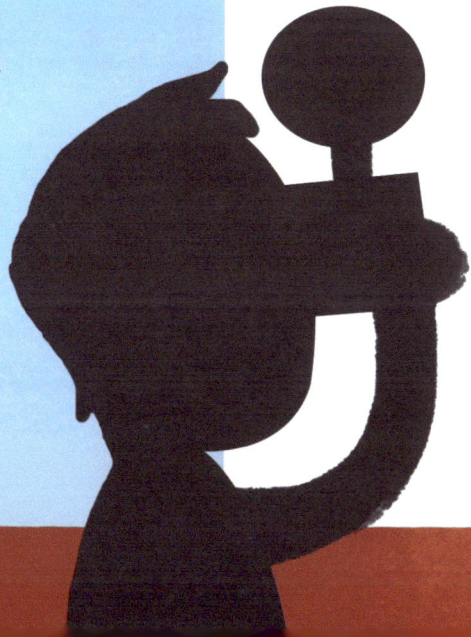

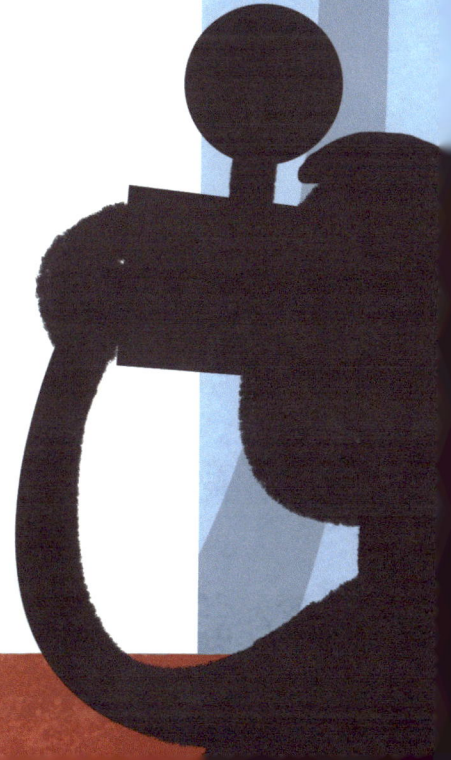

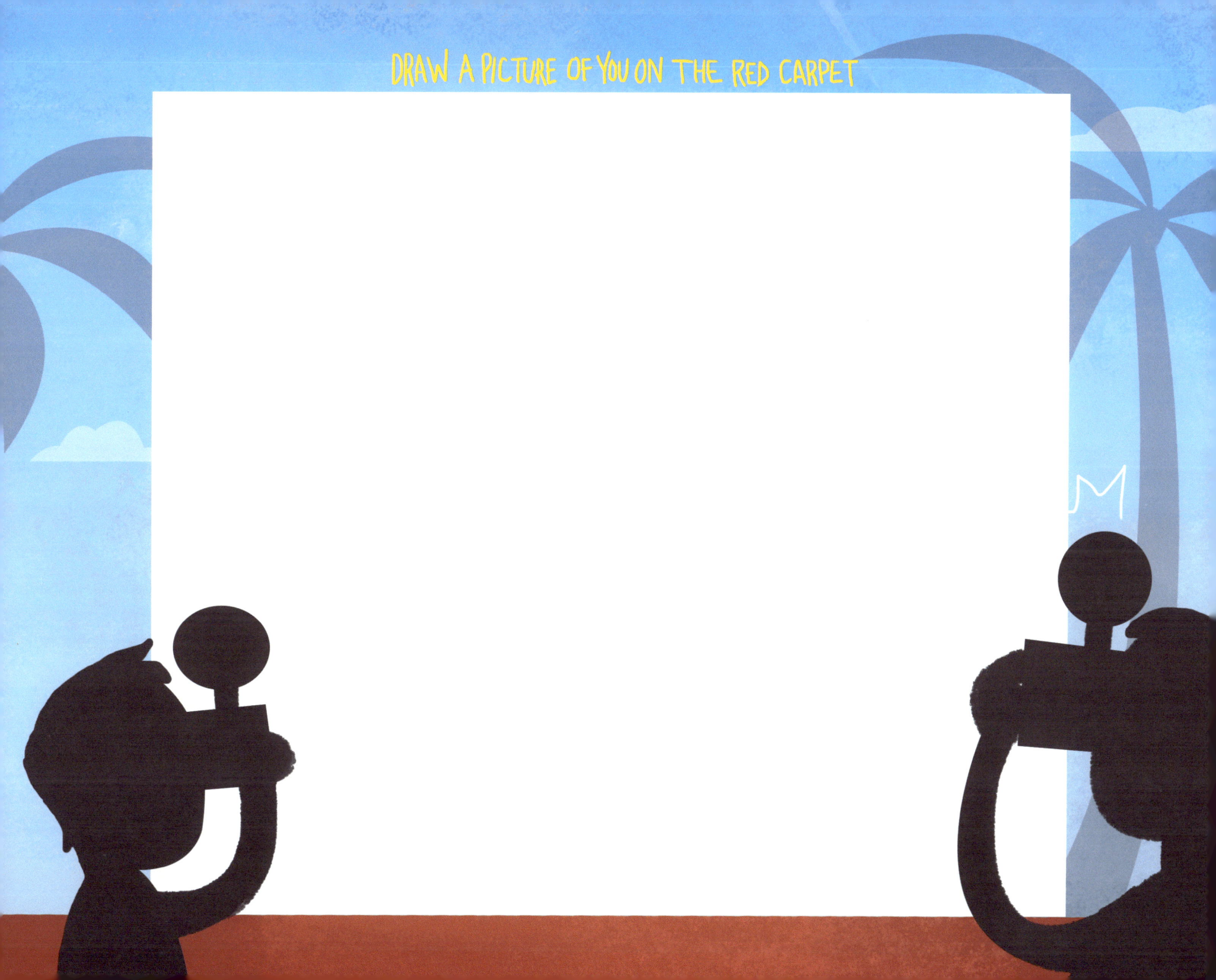

MEMBERS OF MY FAN CLUB

Friends   Family   Visitors

Draw Or Paste A Picture

MEMBERS OF MY ENTOURAGE

Doctors   Nurses   Other People at the Hospital

V.I.P.
CREDITS

Be proud of the amazing things you have accomplished!
Post this list on your wall and add to it everyday.

1. I stayed overnight in the hospital!

2.

3.

4.

5.

6.

7.

8.

9.

10.

GET TO KNOW SOME OTHER STARS OF THE HOSPITAL

Interview members of your growing entourage and draw them in the stars.

Some might be stars you see everyday, or some you just met.

Name:

Job at the hospital:

The work this person does:

What is his/her favorite thing to wear?

I'd also like to know:

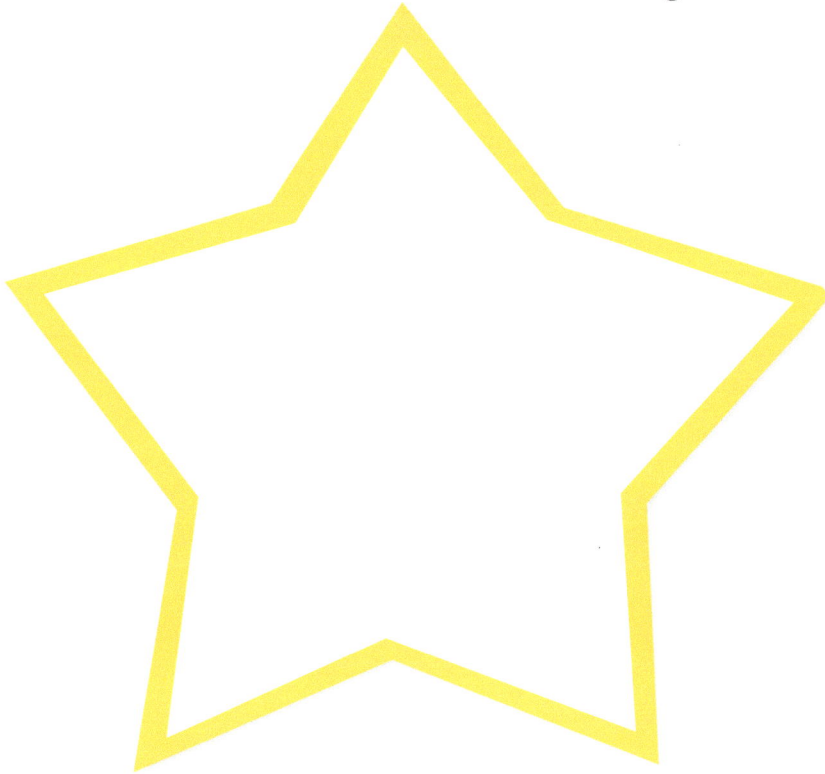

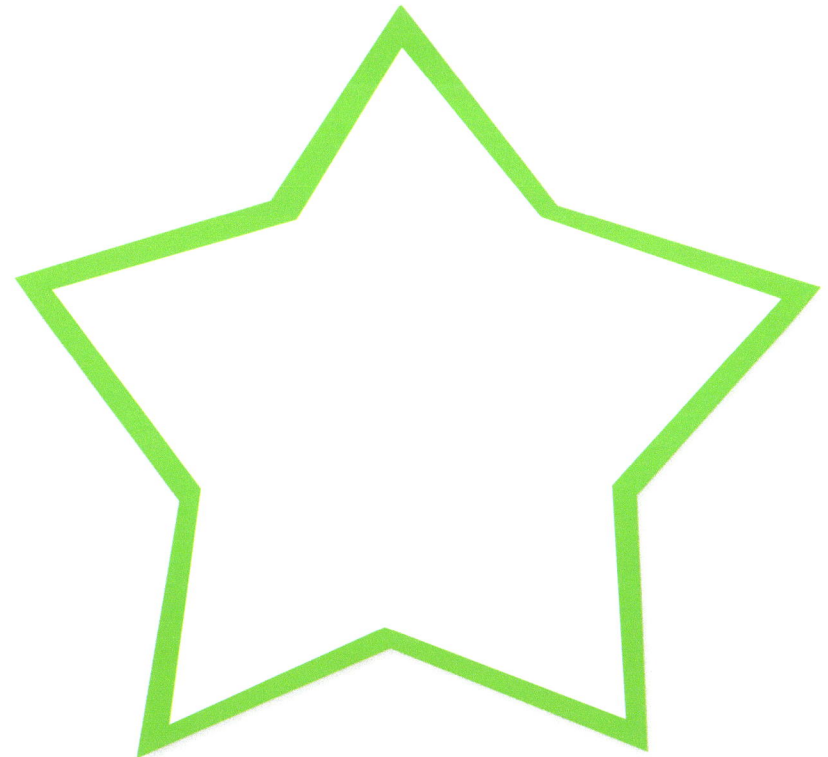

Name:

Job at the hospital:

The work this person does:

What is his/her favorite Disney movie?

I'd also like to know:

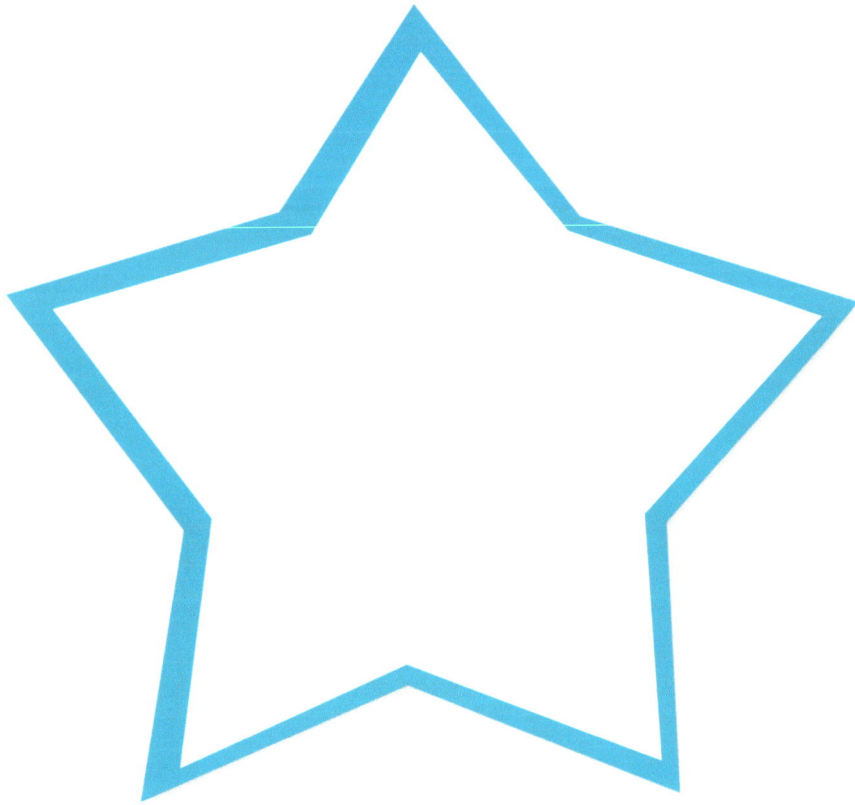

Name:

Job at the hospital:

The work this person does:

What kind of animal would he/she like as a pet?

I'd also like to know:

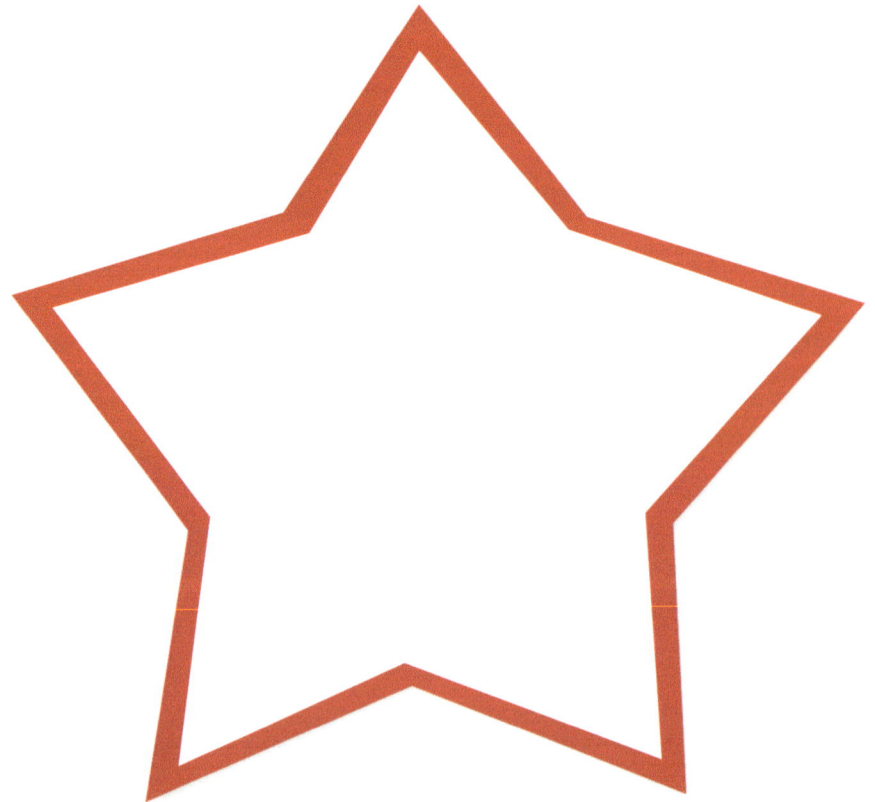

Name:

Job at the hospital:

The work this person does:

What was his/her favorite subject in school?

I'd also like to know:

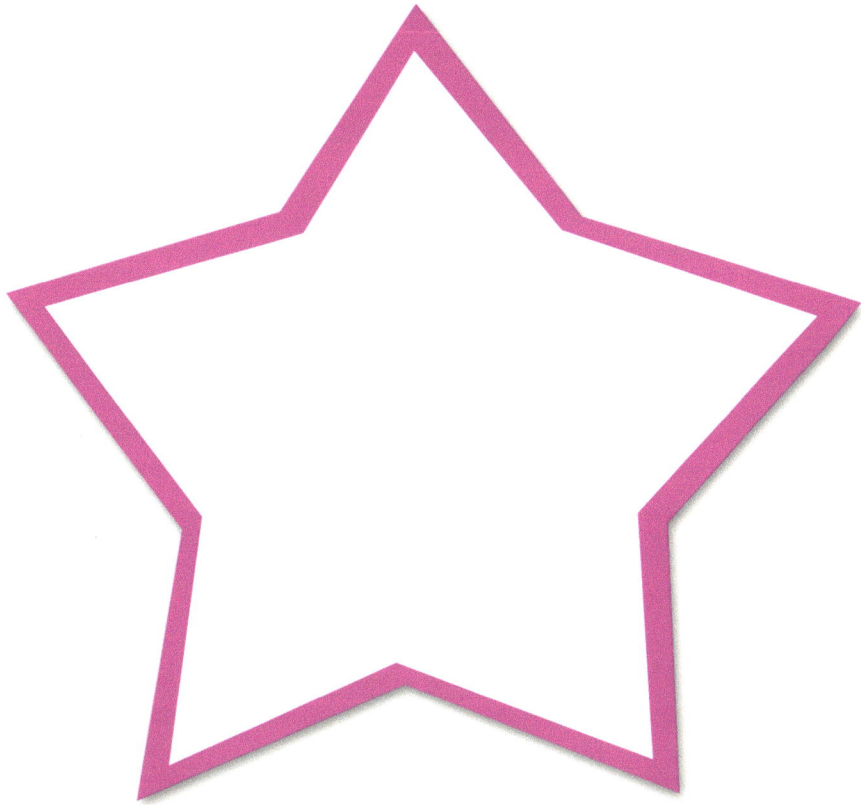

Name:

Job at the hospital:

The work this person does:

What is his/her favorite game to play?

I'd also like to know:

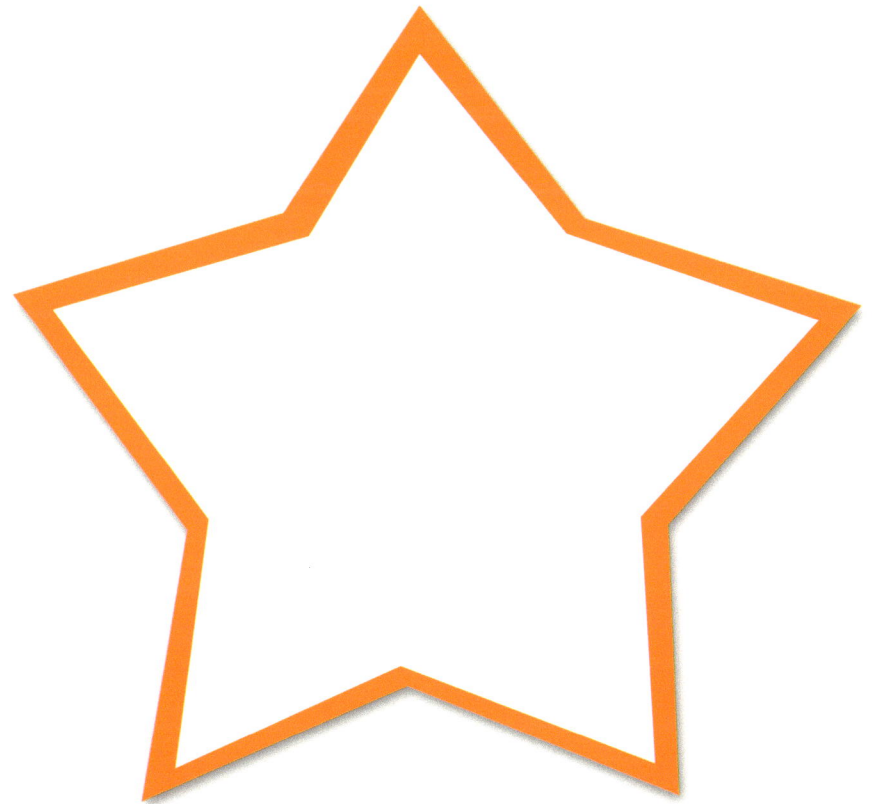

Name:

Job at the hospital:

The work this person does:

How many brothers and sisters does he/she have?

I'd also like to know:

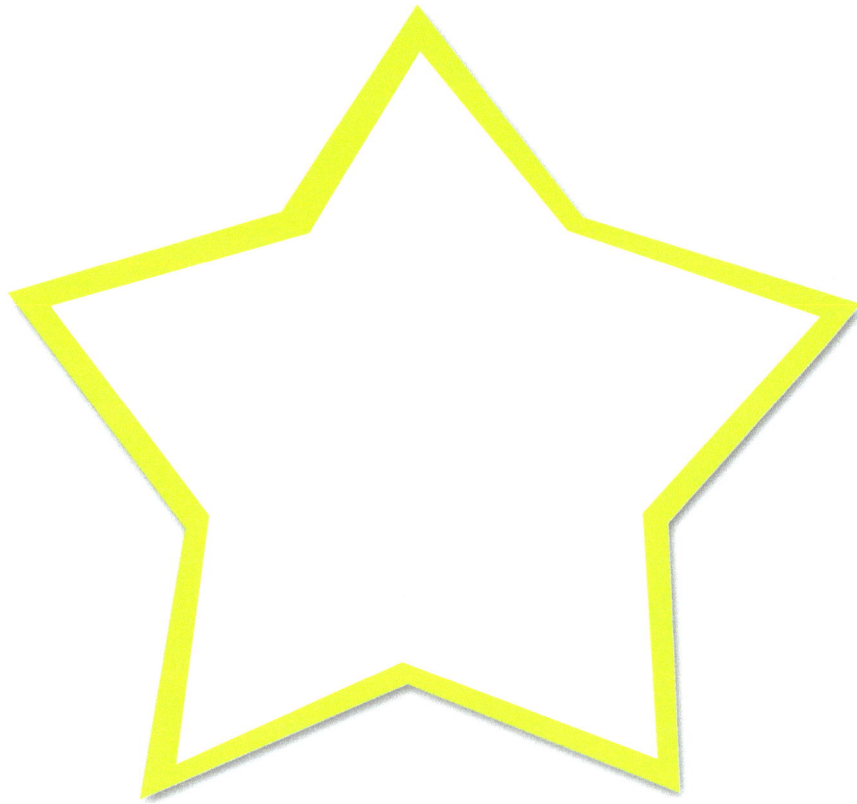

Name:

Job at the hospital:

The work this person does:

Where would he/she go on a dream vacation?

I'd also like to know:

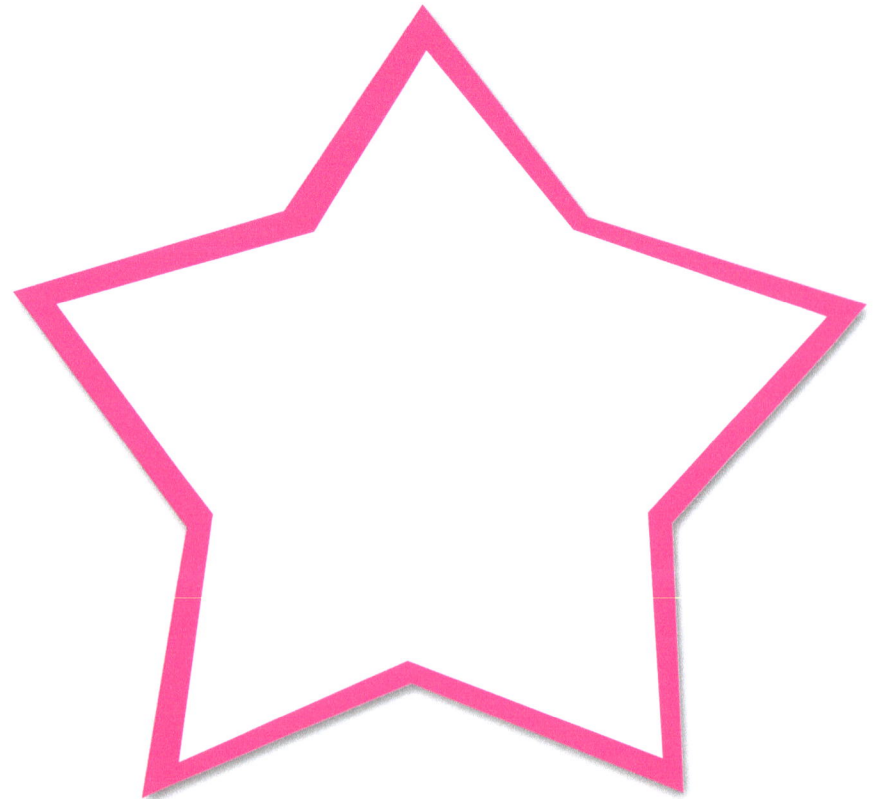

Name:

Job at the hospital:

The work this person does:

What is his/her favorite season?

I'd also like to know:

HALL OF FAME

Collect autographs from other celebrities!
Anyone you meet in the hospital can sign here!

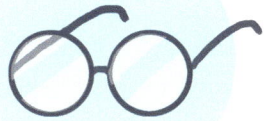

Someone who wears glasses

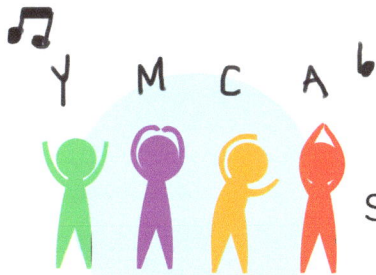

Someone who has black socks

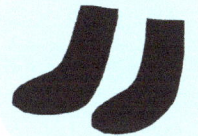

Y M C A

Someone who can do the 'YMCA' dance

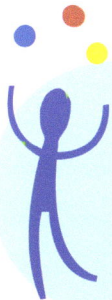

Someone who likes roller coasters

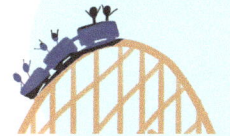

Someone who can juggle

Someone who has a cat

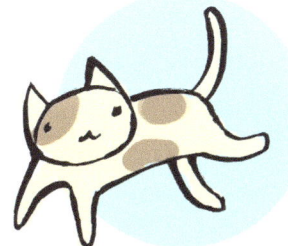

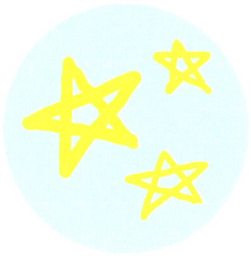

Someone who can sing 'Twinkle Twinkle Little Star' while spinning around

Someone whose favorite color is the same as yours

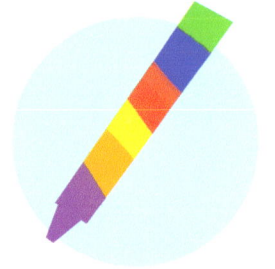

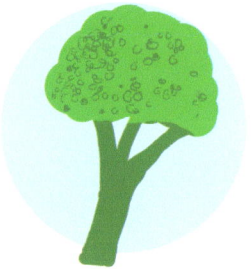

Someone who is a vegetarian

Someone who had a childhood teddy bear

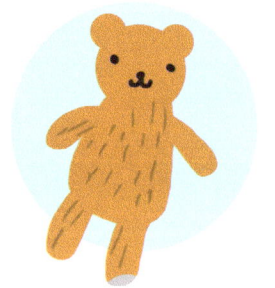

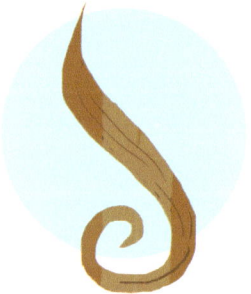

Someone with brown hair

Someone who has been out of the country

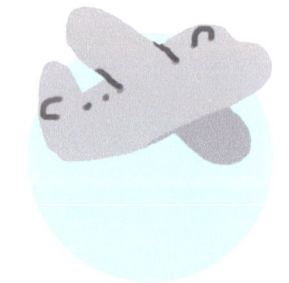

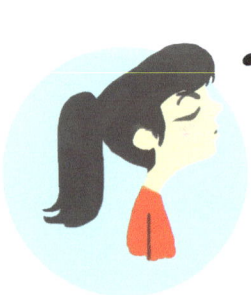

Someone who can whistle

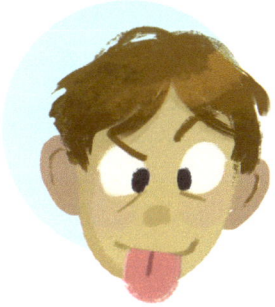

Someone who can make a silly face

Someone who can talk like Donald Duck

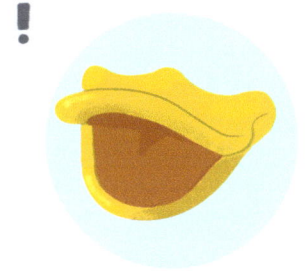

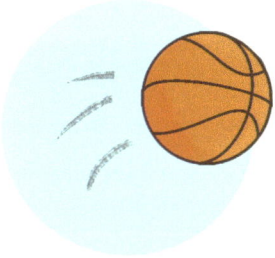

Someone who plays basketball

Someone who is wearing purple

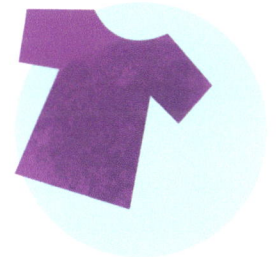

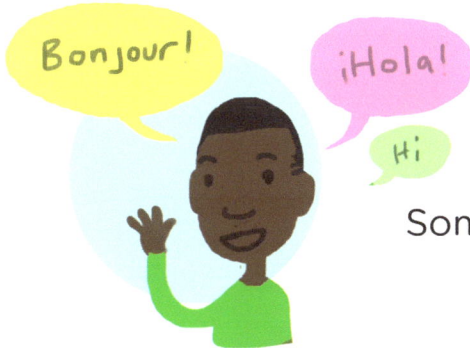

Someone who can speak more than one language

Someone who has been in a school play

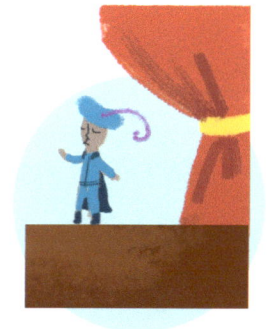

V.I.P. IMPORTANT MEMOS

FOR MY ENTOURAGE

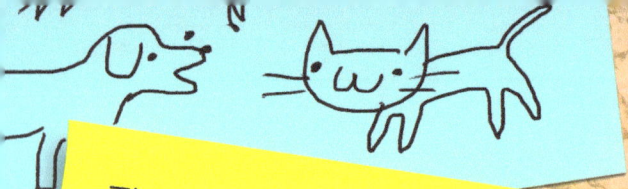

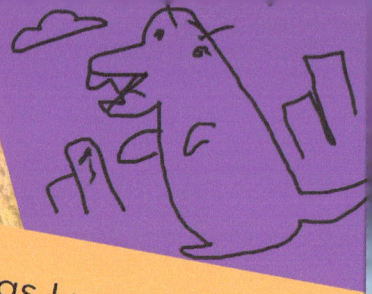

Things I want my entourage to know today are:

Questions I have:

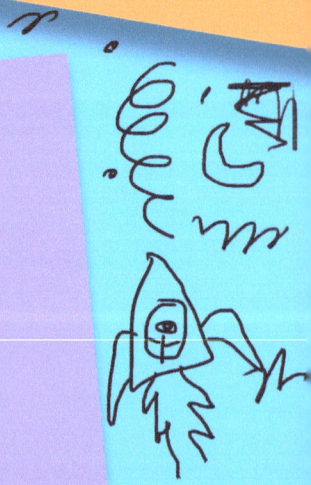

Things I want my entourage to know today are:

Questions I have:

Things I want my entourage to know today are:

Questions I have:

Things I want my entourage to know today are:

Questions I have:

Things I want my entourage to know today are:

Questions I have:

THE V.I.P. HAS A VERY IMPORTANT QUESTION FOR YOU

V.I.P. HAS
A QUESTION

V.I.P. HAS
A QUESTION

Cut out and fold to make a standing sign

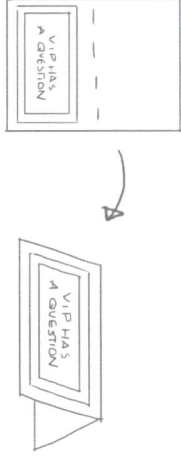

Use this sign whenever you have a question for your entourage

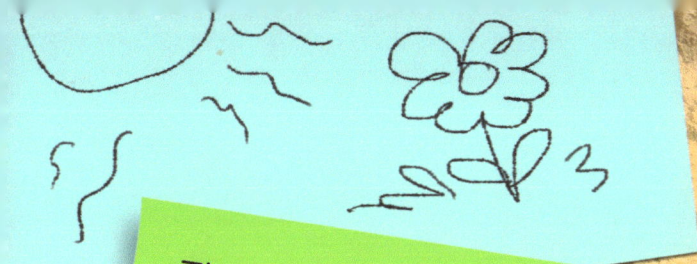

Things I want my entourage to know today are:

Questions I have:

Things I want my entourage to know today are:

Questions I have:

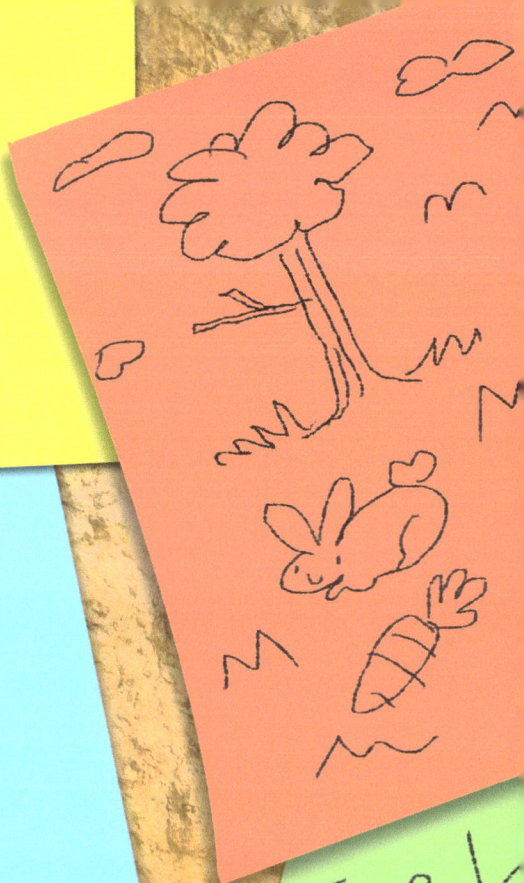

Things I want my entourage to know today are:

Questions I have:

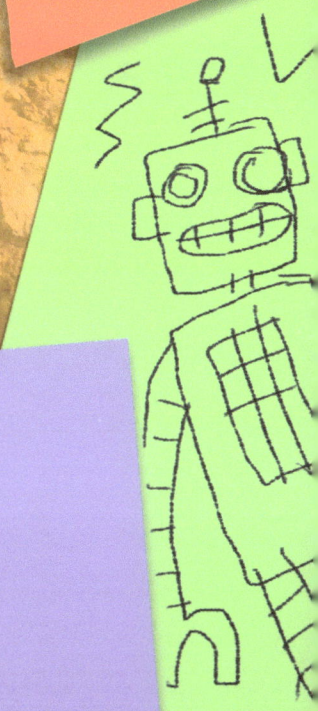

Things I want my entourage to know today are:

Questions I have:

Things I want my entourage to know today are:

Questions I have:

Things I want my entourage to know today are:

Questions I have:

Write A Screenplay

When you get to a different color ask a member
of your entourage to help you with the next part of the story!

Once upon a time there was

_____

_____

_____

Then one day

_____

_____

_____

And then, something really funny happened

_____

_____

_____

Then something unbelievable occurred

_____

_____

_____

_____

But luckily, everything worked out when

_____

_____

_____

_____

_____

_____

THE END

NOW SHOWING

Draw a poster for your movie and share it with your entourage!

The V.i.p. Times

V.I.P. PRESS!

ASK MEMBERS OF YOUR ENTOURAGE AND FAN CLUB TO WRITE WORDS AND PHRASES THAT DESCRIBE YOU!

COSTUME DESIGNS

Create some fun superheroes!
Ask a member of your entourage to help with the parts in red

NAME:

POWERS:

DRAW A PICTURE OF THEM IN THEIR COSTUME

NAME:

POWERS:

DESCRIBE WHAT THEY SHOULD WEAR:

DRAW A PICTURE OF THEM IN THEIR COSTUME

POW

NAME:

POWERS:

DESCRIBE WHAT THEY SHOULD WEAR:

DRAW A PICTURE OF THEM IN THEIR COSTUME

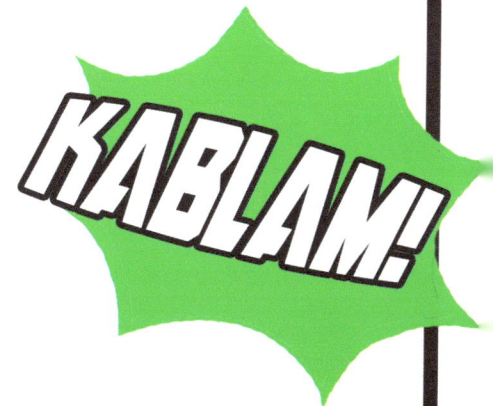

NAME:

POWERS:

DRAW A PICTURE OF THEM IN THEIR COSTUME

KABLAM!

you and your

Channel your inner Paparazzi and take some photos!

This is me dancing with:

This is me making a Thumbs-Up sign with:

entourage

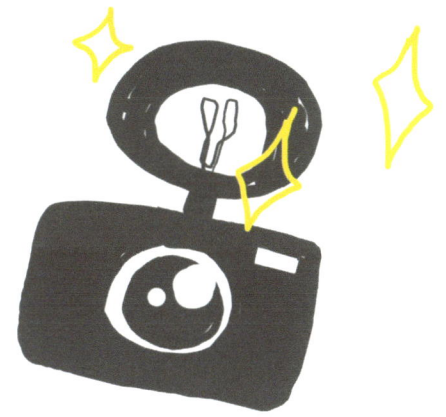

This is me with:

Making our silliest faces!

This is me with:

Acting as if we just won
a MILLION dollars!

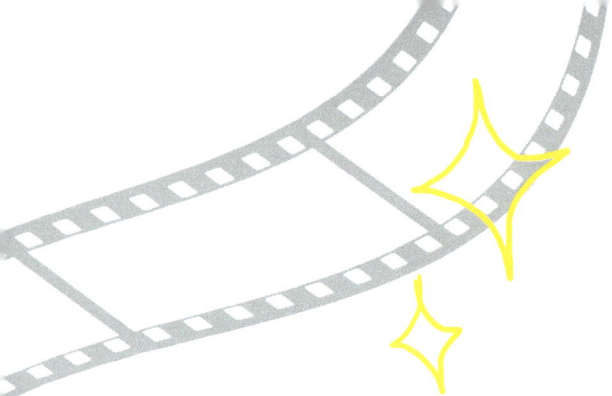

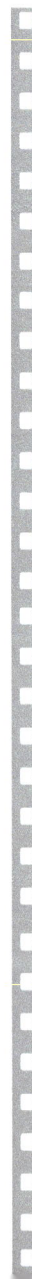

This is me with:

Posing for a magazine cover!

This is me with:

We are:

Give your own personalized awards to people who make you feel like a Very Important Patient!

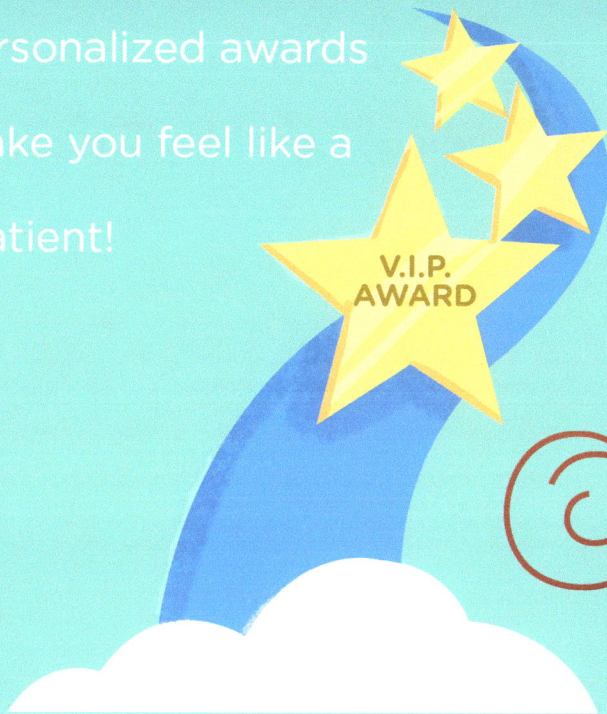

The First Annual

V.I.P. Awards

V.I.P. AWARD

Thank you for being so nice to me!
It makes me feel so good to know you care!

AWARDED TO _____

FROM _____

V.I.P. AWARD

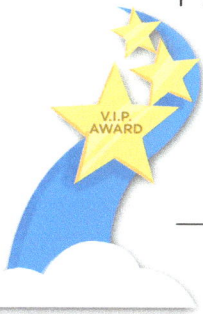

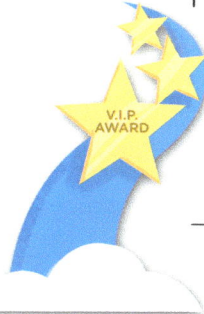

_____
(Official V.I.P. Signature)

Thank you for always making me smile
and brightening my day!

AWARDED TO _____

FROM _____

V.I.P. AWARD

_____
(Official V.I.P. Signature)

Thank you for _____

_____

AWARDED TO _____

FROM _____

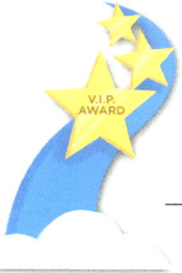

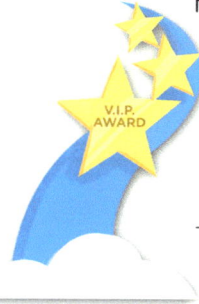

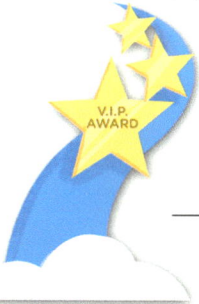

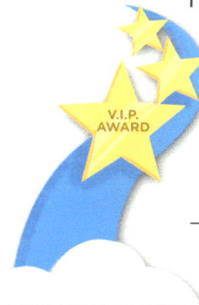

_____
(Official V.I.P. Signature)

Thank you for _____

_____

AWARDED TO _____

FROM _____

_____
(Official V.I.P. Signature)

Thank you for _____

_____

AWARDED TO _____

FROM _____

_____
(Official V.I.P. Signature)

Thank you for _____

_____

AWARDED TO _____

FROM _____

_____
(Official V.I.P. Signature)

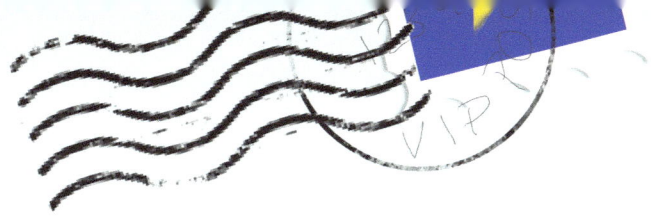

FAN MAIL

Dear V.I.P.

I was wondering what are some things that always make you laugh?

_____

_____

_____

_____

Dear V.I.P.

Tell me about a time when you felt brave!

_____

_____

_____

_____

Dear V.I.P.

What do you do when you're scared of something?

_____

_____

_____

What helps to make you not so scared?

_____

_____

_____

_____

Dear V.I.P.

What is the hardest thing about being in the hospital?

_____

_____

_____

_____

What are some things that make it better?

_____

_____

_____

_____

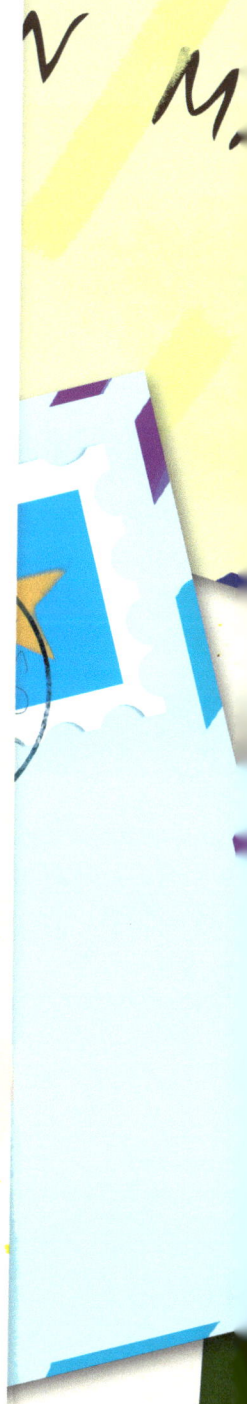

Dear V.I.P.

I'm a huge fan! I'm in the hospital for the same reason as you. Do you have any advice for me to make it less scary? You can draw pictures too. I love those!

Dear fan,

I want to tell you about: _____

_____

_____

This is what happened: _____

_____

_____

Some questions I had were: _____

_____

_____

If this happens to you, you should know: _____

_____

_____

I felt: _____

_____

_____

I thought: _____

_____

_____

Turn the page →

Here's a picture about it for you:

iggest Fan
23 Road
VIP City

Visit our website to contribute your stories
and see what other V.I.P.'s like you have posted!
www.viphospitalproductions.org

Share your fan mail
with your entourage!

www.ingramcontent.com/pod-product-compliance
Lightning Source LLC
Chambersburg PA
CBHW041552030426

42336CB00004B/54